One Poke, Two Pokes, Three… This is Not a Joke!

N'Jhari Jackson

One Poke, Two Pokes, Three

Copyright © 2017 N'Jhari Jackson

All rights reserved.

ISBN-10:1987439775
ISBN-13:9781987439779

One Poke, Two Pokes, Three

DEDICATION

This children's book is dedicated to all kids who have experienced 'One Poke, Two Pokes, Three…,"
or wake-up every day with a 'permanent scar.'
May you laugh until you pee your pants and cry until you smile!

Your One Poke, Two Pokes, Three Buddy, NJ

One Poke, Two Pokes, Three

One Poke, Two Pokes, Three

CONTENTS

	Acknowledgments	i
1	One Poke	1
2	Two Pokes	Pg. 5
3	Three Pokes	Pg. 7
4	Yo! This is not a joke!	Pg. 11
5	What Kids Should Be Doing…	Pg. 14
5	Meet Hailey Bankhead	Pg. 18
6	Meet Bailey Rhodes	Pg. 22
7	Meet the Juggernaut	Pg. 29
8	About the Author	Pg. 35

One Poke, Two Pokes, Three

ACKNOWLEDGMENTS

In all do, in all I will become, in all that I am, I acknowledge God as my Lord and Savior! I thank Dick Vitale's **V Foundation** for its tireless research efforts in finding a cure for pediatric cancer. Though they've experienced one poke, two pokes, three…, Hailey Bankhead and the Princess Hailey Bankhead Foundation along with Bailey Rhodes' Project Code Gray give back to kids with cancer and other long term illnesses. I am humbled and forever grateful for their efforts in helping to ease the frustrations, anxiety that go with every poke, scan, hospitalization, and physical manifestations of fighting childhood illnesses. Thank you to the many organizations, donors, volunteers, scientist who help to offset the mere 4% funding for Pediatric Cancer Research.

Proverbs 3: 6

In all your ways acknowledge him, and he will make straight your paths.

One Poke, Two Pokes, Three

1

ONE POKE

Woke up no longer me looking at bright orange shirts on he, she, and even Brea. Thus, making me a, we. I got a team strangely I didn't recruit. In and out of sleep maybe it's just a fluke.

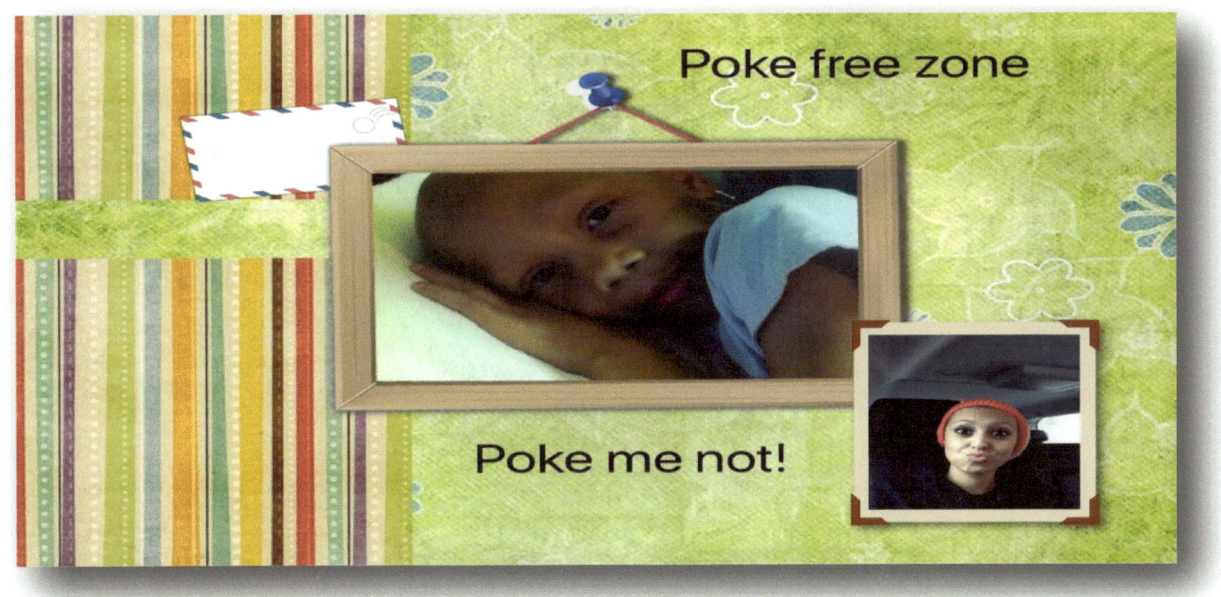

The world is moving fast like a race, feels like I'm coming in last. By the way, how did I get in this itchy cast? I catch a glimpse of dad, newly stamped crow's feet on the side of his eyes; hardened cheeks tell he's mad. Thinking to myself was I really that bad.

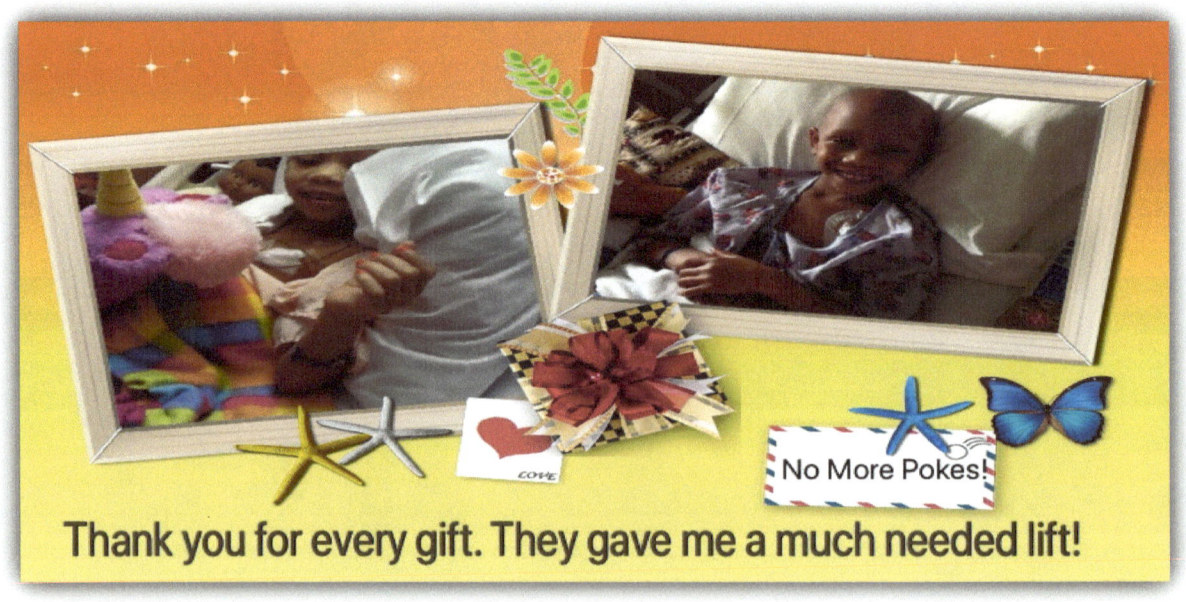

2

TWO POKES

Tiny am I in this hospital bed; stuffed animals galore brought so much joy. It's getting a little crowded, please no more. Laying here thinking life's not fair realizing this O' childhood O' mine is not a crystal stair; refusing to look in the mirror eyes parched to an empty glare.

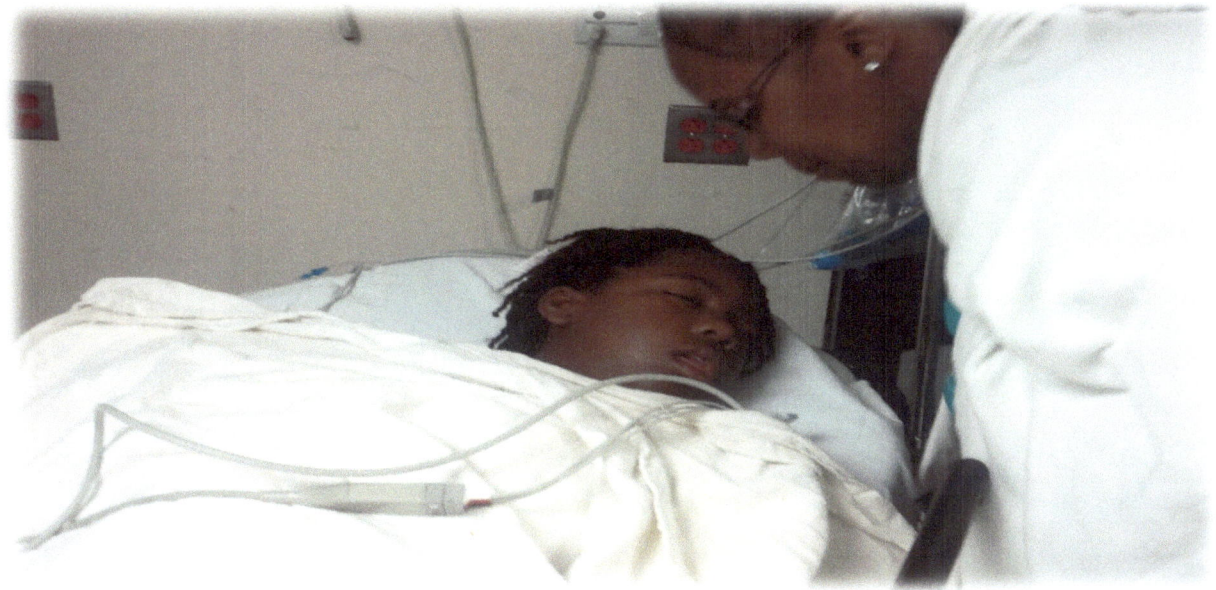

Tubes and lines engulf me; somebody, anybody please help me. Mommy says, "she got me! She'll never leave me because He made us a, we." He bared the burden for you, me and now we. Okay then, why do they keep poking me and only me, not we, she or Thee? I guess that's the way it must be!

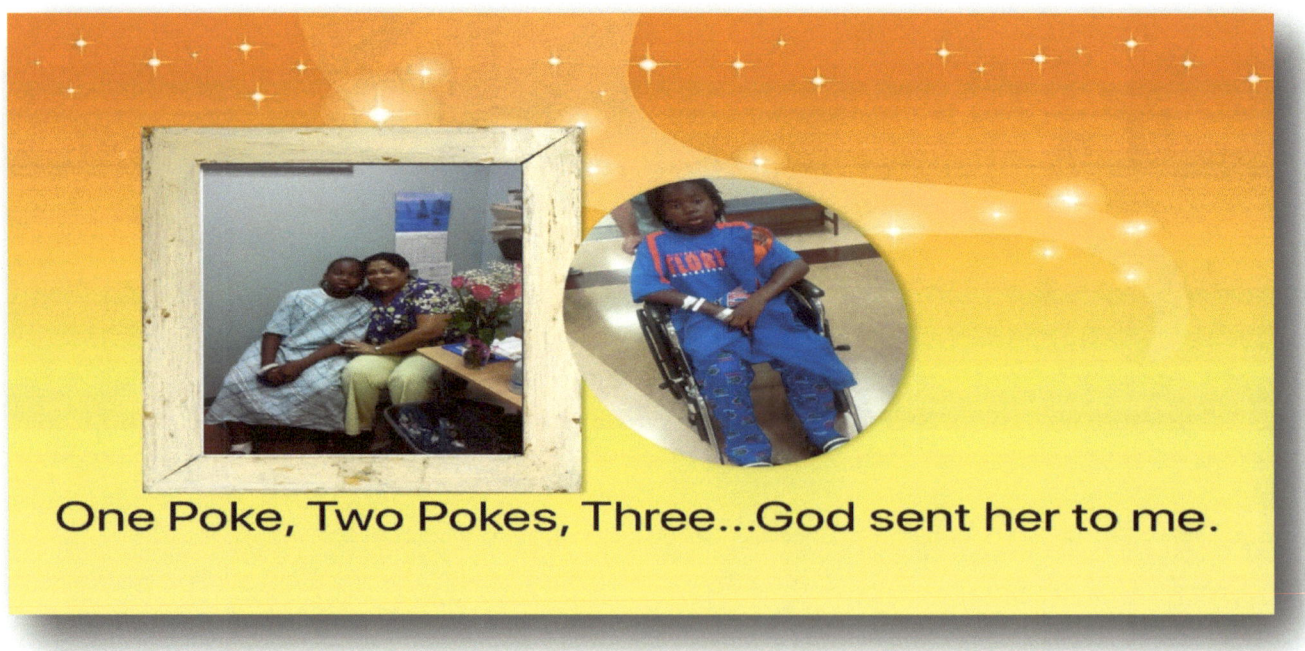

One Poke, Two Pokes, Three...God sent her to me.

3

THREE POKES

One poke, two pokes, three… Yo! This is not a joke. Did dude think I was sleeping? Yo! I'm very much woke. Fluid flows through my veins like napalm hitting my organs like a bomb. The boy down hall his name was John. Liquid napalm tho' powerful enough, had him feeling O' so roughed up constantly hurling stuff up. Quiet so loud, I hear the tears fall; priest name Father Paul says, "he's gone."

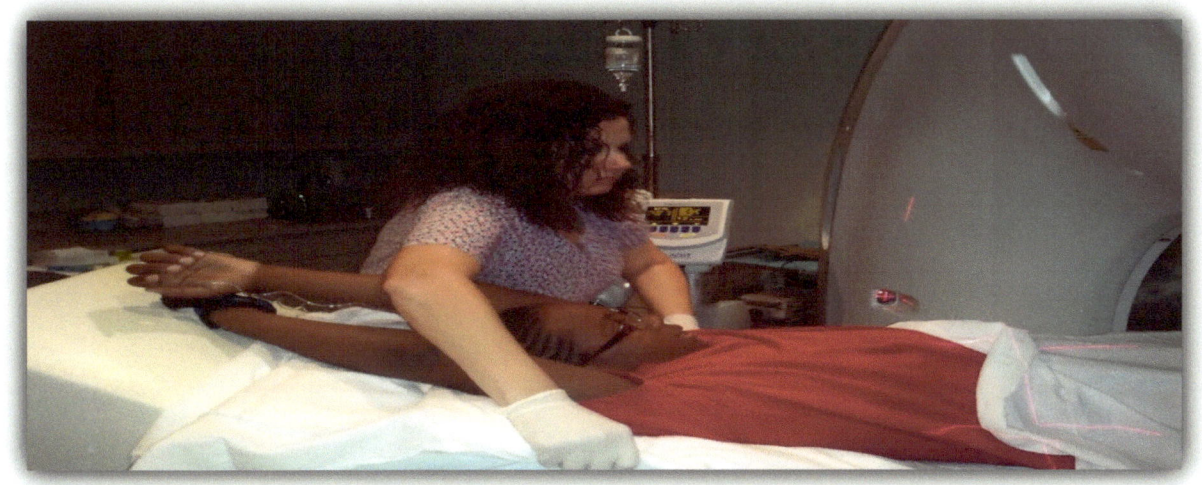

I ask myself, what did he do so wrong? Look at me I got no hair, bones bare people stare asking myself, "Where did I go?" Clothes too big, mom bought me a wig. People smile, I smile too. Well, at least on the outside I do! Skin fried, eyes dried, grandma cried, and the nurse keeps saying, "I'm adorable" as she cleans my mess. I don't think she's seen the stains from the puke on her dress.

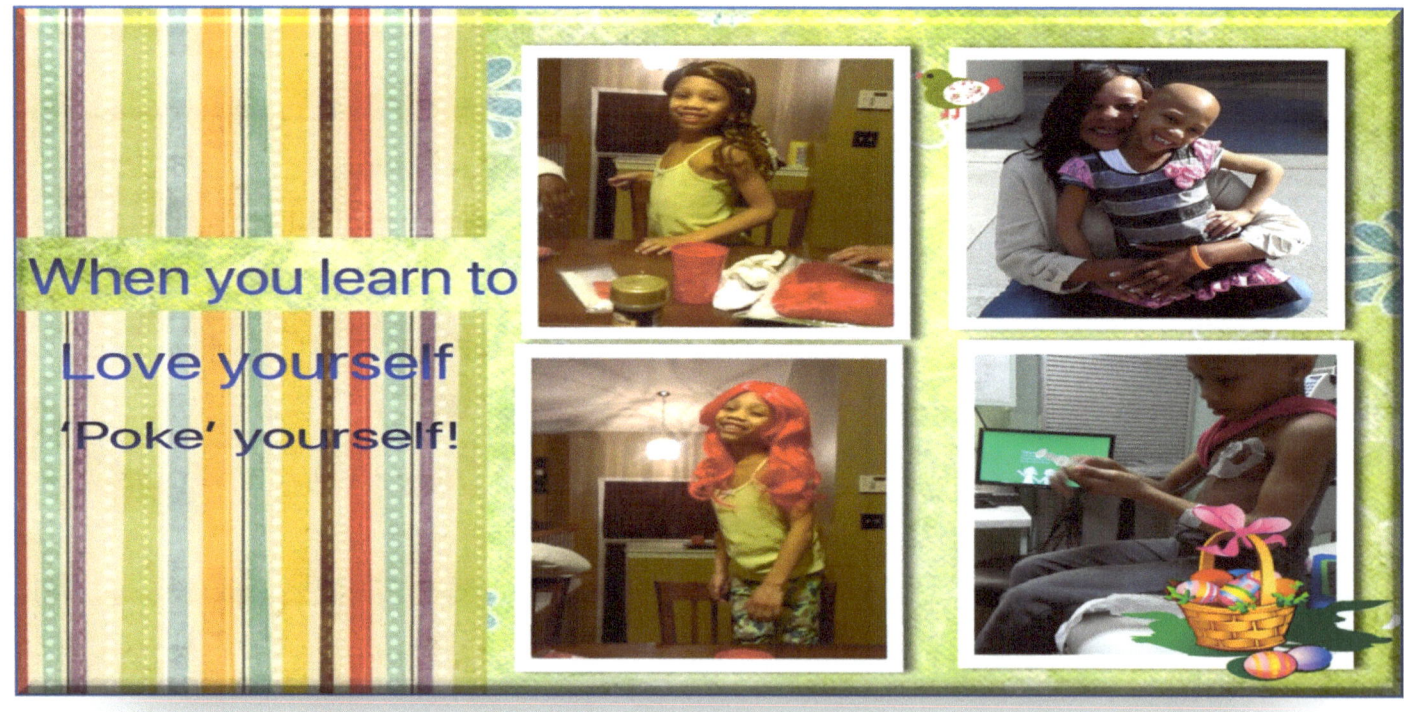

Trying to take it all in stride substituting scan tables for a carnival ride. Complete with lights, lasers, and even remote control Tasers. Handing me headphones as she speaks to me on a microphone, thinking please, "I just really want to go home." Now, "Stay real still," she commands like it's no big deal. I'm thinking, "Only, if looks could kill."

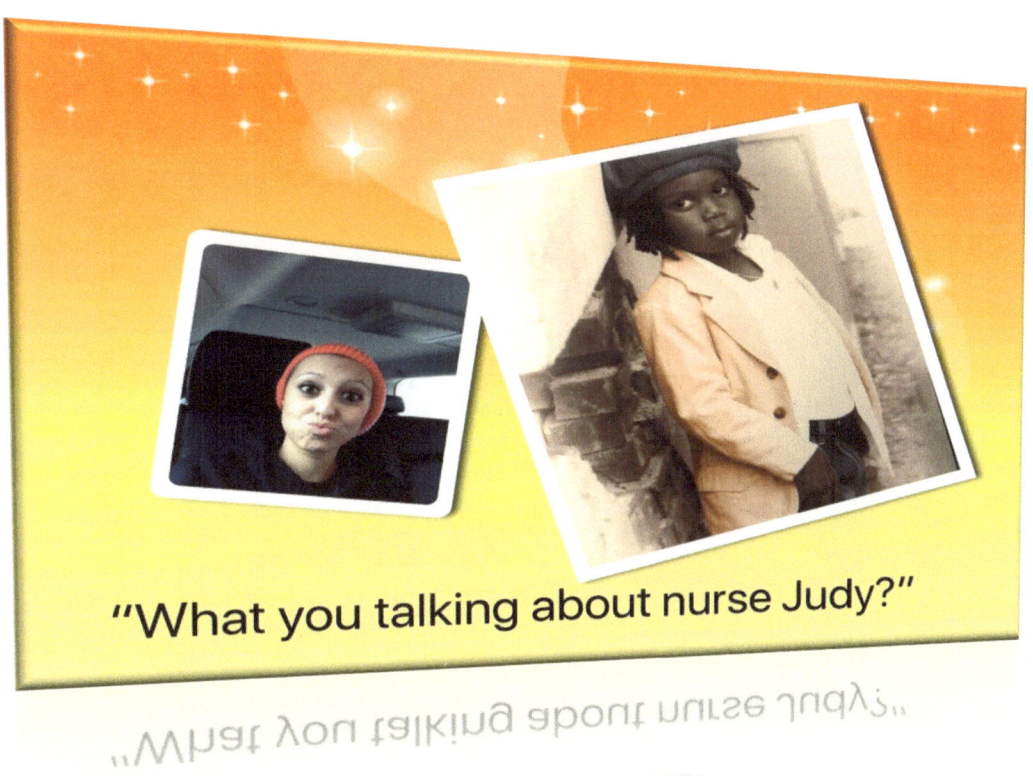

"What you talking about nurse Judy?"

One Poke, Two Pokes, Three

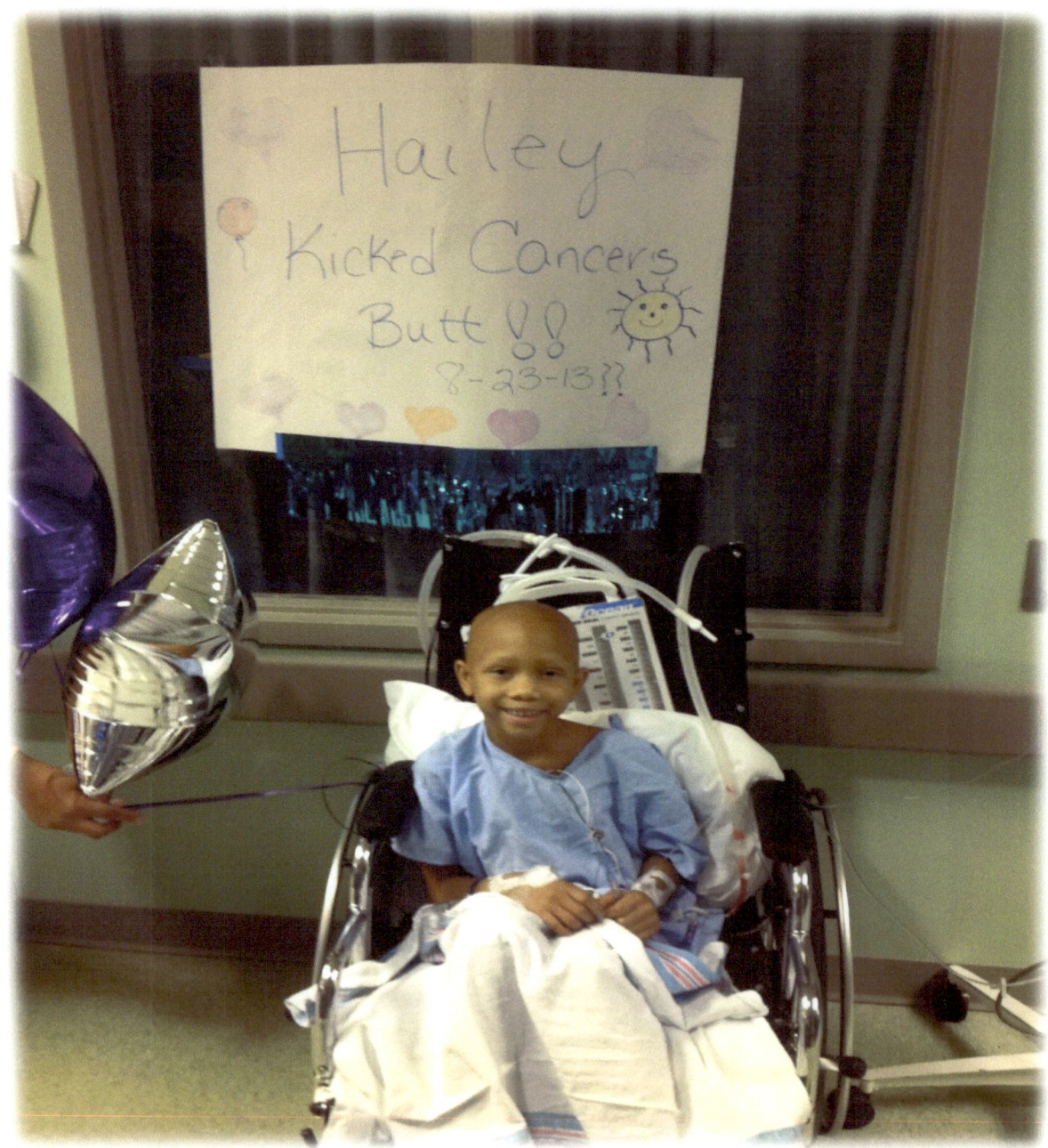

4

YO! THIS IS NOT A JOKE!

I may be a fool. Why you ask? I miss being at school. Tho' kids can be rude,

some are really cool. I'll take my chances just get me out of this hospital room.

Chemicals got me feeling drained, some days can't remember my dog's name.

Now, that's a shame! Medically, they call it "fog brain," as my body wanes.

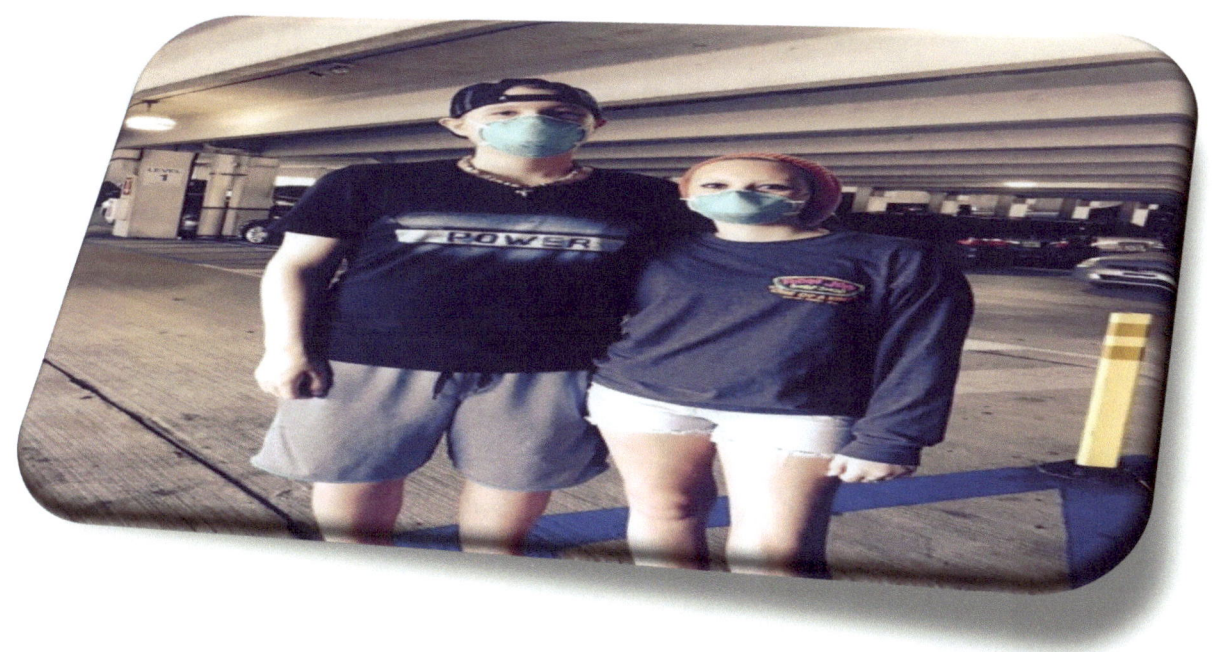

Hiding my face with a paper mask not sure which is worse, this itchy cast or this awful mask. Did I mention, everyone has good intentions asking, "How do you feel?" Let's see, taking pills that can kill and I'm supposed to be chill, smile and swallow these pills, look-up and say, "I'm doing just swell." As the nurse patiently waits, she's armed with a weapon that impales.

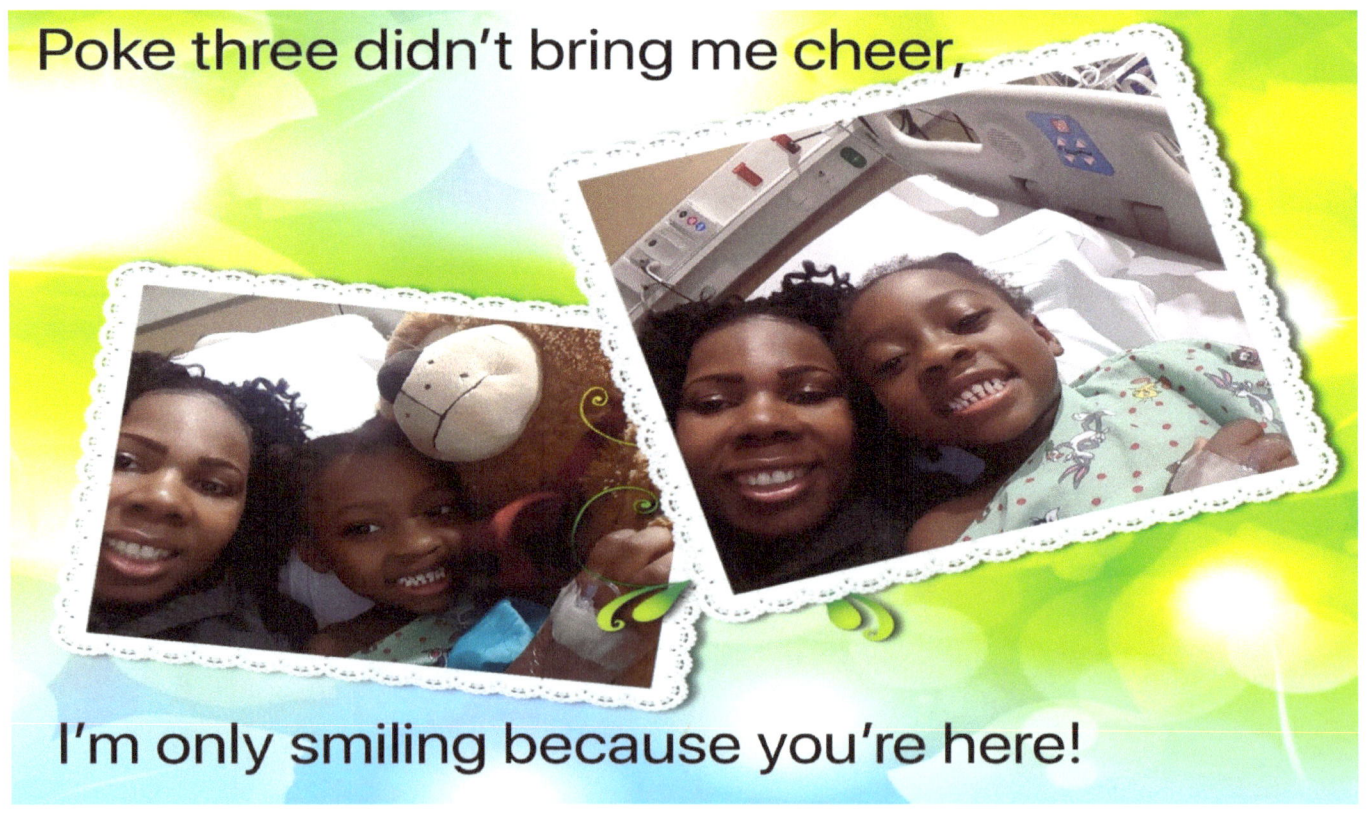

But hey, I perk up for you, she, and even the guy with aunt Bee just so they'd hurry up and flee and let me be. Besides, there's puke waiting to leave me and gladly they'll turn their backs and I set-it-free. No time to say, "excuse me!"

Doctor says, "Sweetie get some rest," but how can I when they keep poking at my chest wishing I had a bullet proof vest. 12-gauge needles, Lasers, beams, and napalm bombs going off in my arms. Nurse says, "honey, stay calm." Call me crazy maybe even a little lazy, tell me that again and she'll be pushing up daisies…. Well, maybe!

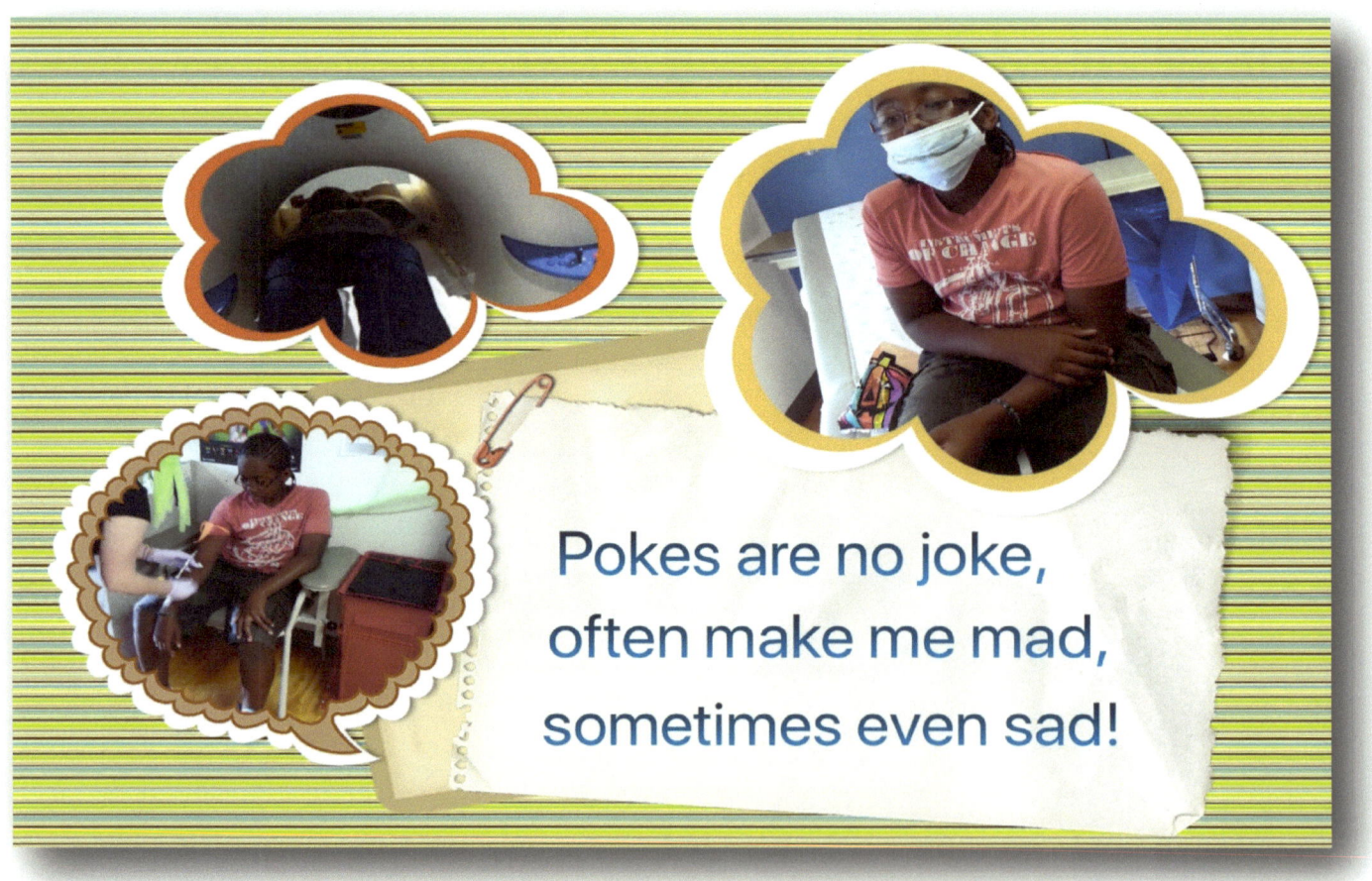

Pokes are no joke, often make me mad, sometimes even sad!

When kids are not worried about 'One Poke, Two Pokes, Three,' we are free to be who we were wonderfully made to be...

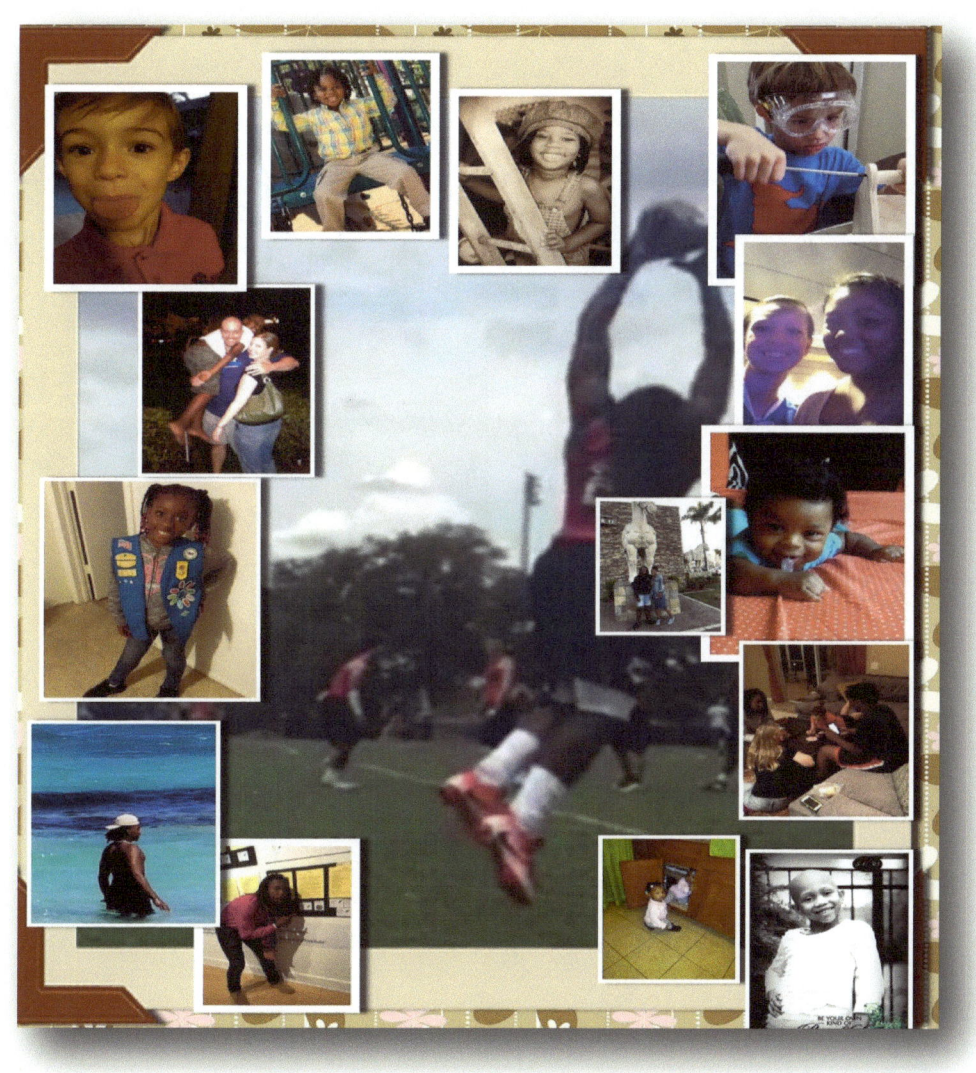

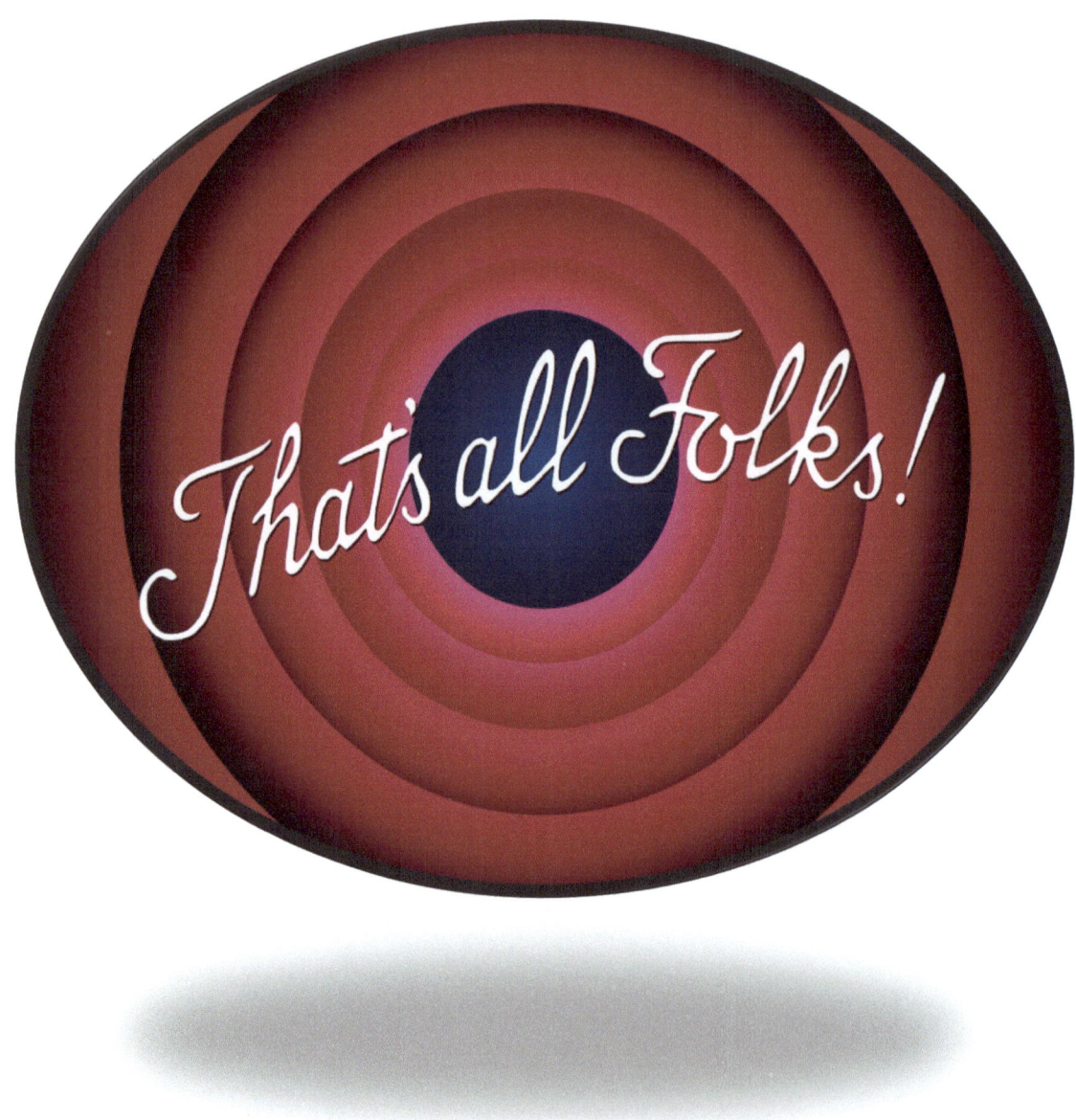

NOT QUITE…

MEET MY ONE POKE, TWO POKES, THREE BUDDIES… SCOUT'S HONOR, YOU'RE GOING TO ENJOY MEETING THEM!

MEET HAILEY BANKHEAD

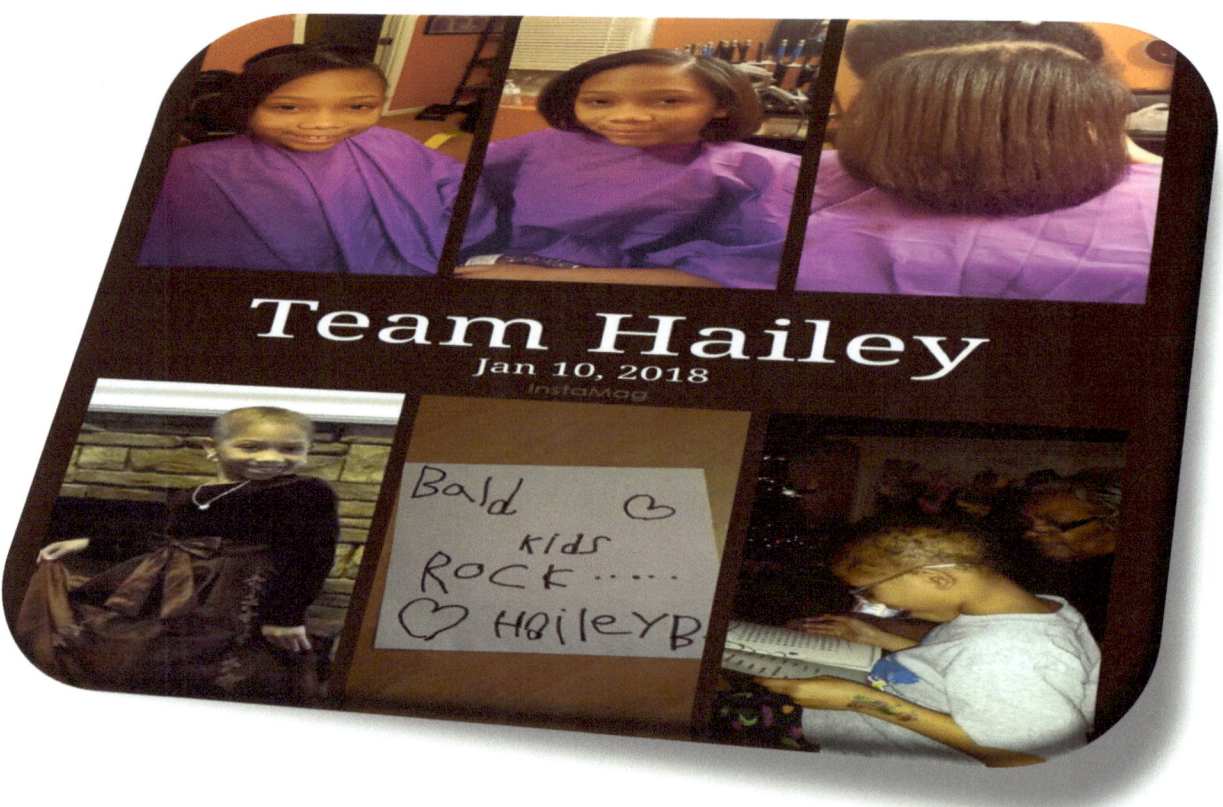

Hailey is one of the millions of kids afflicted with a childhood illness that subjects her to One Poke, Two Pokes, Three. According Hailey's mom, Heather Bankhead, "being diagnosed with cancer is a very scary experience for any child, hard to understand, painful to endure and challenging to cope." She goes on to introduce readers her daughter to, Hailey

Bankhead who was diagnosed with stage IV Wilms Tumor on January 15, 2013, at the age of 5. It later spread to her lungs. Hailey's journey consisted of 30 days of radiation and 7 months of chemotherapy. Hailey had to have one of her kidney's and lymph nodes removed. As of August 22, 2013, Hailey is in remission. Hailey's maintenance care is done every three months which consist of One Poke, Two Pokes, Three and a full body scan.

Despite the routine treatments and hospital/doctor visits, Hailey lives a normal life as a "Little Diva." She enjoys going to school and being interactive with her classmates. Her hobbies include: shopping and cheerleading. You can also find Hailey playing outside with her friends making-up lost time. She loves to laugh and tell jokes. She is a people person and loves making people feel better. Hailey is also the spokesperson for the Hailey Bankhead Foundation, Inc. The author, N'Jhari Jackson found out Hailey's condition through a family member who lives in California. Hailey was hospitalized in Atlanta, GA while N'Jhari and his mom in Tampa, FL. N'Jhari through his Pajama Buddy Voyage Mission took it upon himself with the help of his mom to drive to Atlanta to personally deliver a special Pajama Buddy Drab Bag and Buddy to Hailey the day after the removal of her kidney. N'Jhari told Hailey at the time, "I am filling a gap for auntie Kerri (California) and bringing you a smile." N'Jhari was nice enough to bring Pajama Buddies for all the kids in the Unit at Eggleston Children's Hospital. They've been buddies from that point on even joining forces to deliver smiles to kids from Florida to Georgia.

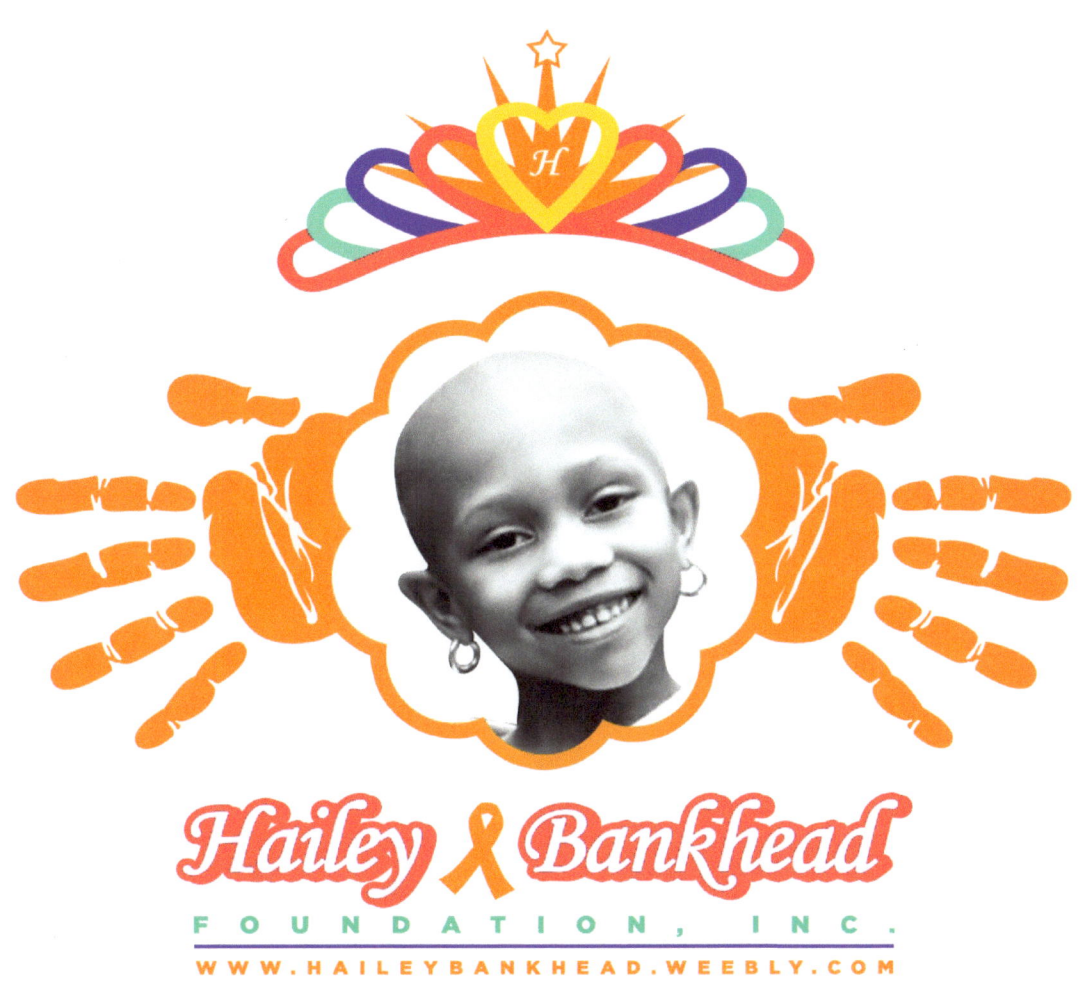

N'Jhari Jackson

MEET BAILEY RHODES

Bailey though extremely tough and always up for a challenge, being diagnosed with Osteosarcoma was not a welcomed challenge. Though frightening, Bailey was determined to do battle and win! She spent the first half of high school in the rink battling bone cancer, only to rejoin the fight where cancer asked for a rematch. This second round would last the better part of her junior and senior year with leukemia as the opponent.

Bailey says, "I just looked at it (cancer) and my goal was to get out of there (the hospital) because I had a lot of stuff to do; and I kept focused." She was forced to miss more than a year of school with most of that time being spent in the hospital. Despite her time away from the traditional classroom, Bailey still graduated on time with honors. "She's a fighter…a Champion!" Cancer though a tough battle, was no match for a champion. Many around her can attest to a Bailey's "Moving forward, positive outlook on life," ever focused on getting better, getting stronger, and moving-on.

Bailey attest to being a, "control freak." Her needing to be in control of her situation led her question, research, and understand information pertaining to not only her pediatric cancer, but other childhood illnesses and their experience as long term pediatric patients. Her control birthed a project near and dear to her heart, **Code Gray. Code Gray** is a special notebook designed by Bailey to help cancer patients self-advocate and track their progress.

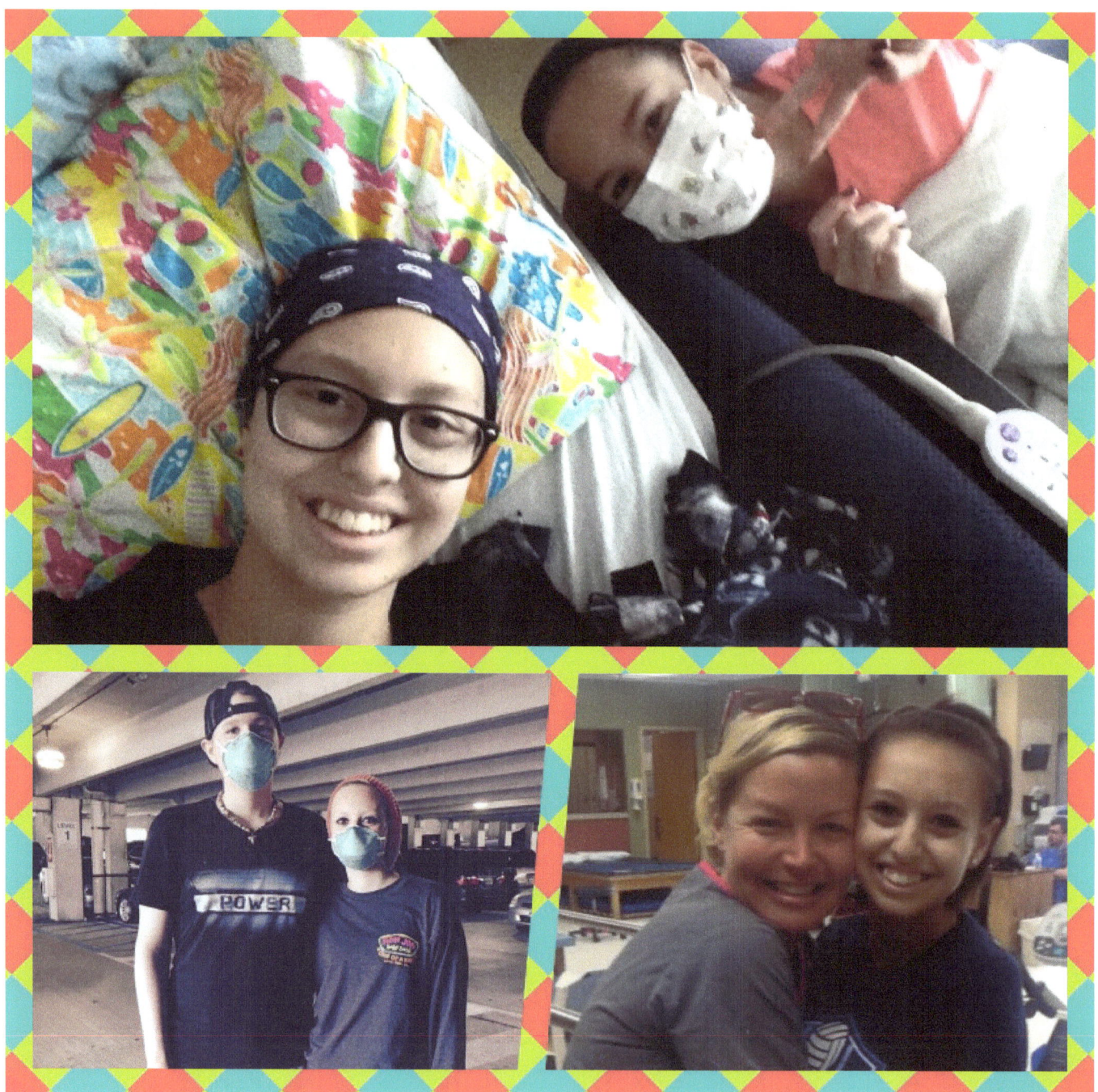

Bailey explains that, "If you are the patient, you are the only constant that's always there. You're the one receiving the medicine; you're the one who knows exactly how it feels and how you react to certain things," Inside each booklet there is a section to help patients keep track of their medication, diet, test results and doctor visits, and even a section to write down questions patients want answered by medical professionals. During her time of treatment and being in-patient, Bailey kept track of her treatments and even caught a medical mistake along the way. Bailey explained, "If I'm getting stuck with the needle, I can ask about the needle'," said Bailey. Bailey was determined to control her One Poke, Two Pokes, Three as best she could by decreasing the chance for mistakes.

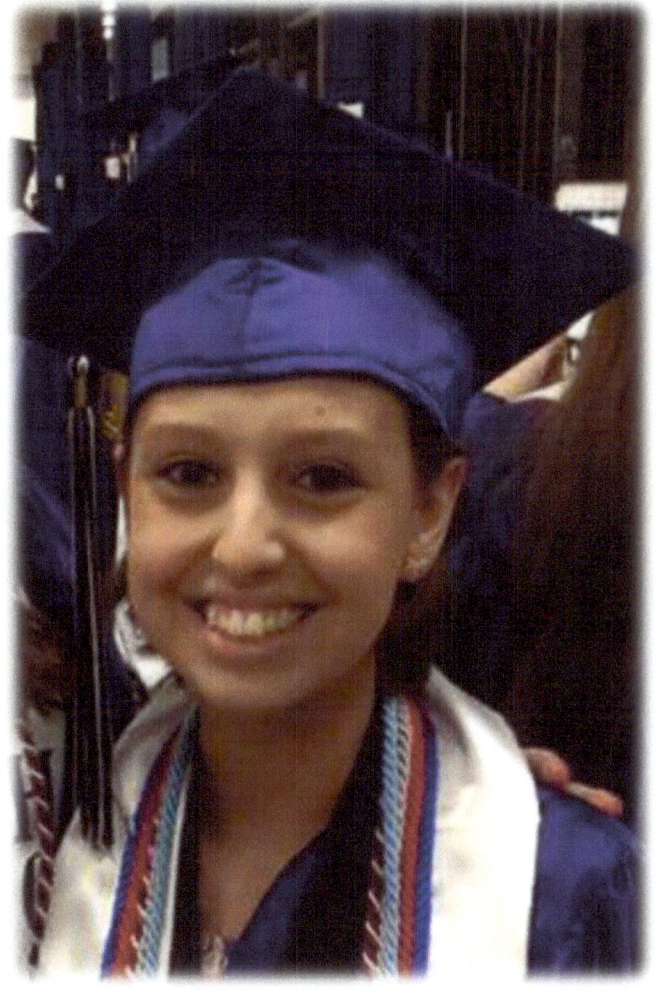

She's advocates other patients to take charge of their treatment and recovery with **Code Gray!** With confidence and surety, Bailey says, "I'm not afraid to speak up for myself. Just because you don't have a medical degree, doesn't mean you don't know what's going on." It is Bailey's hope that **Code Gray** will help other patients realize that even though they're sick, they're not helpless… And that's what a champion sound like, folks!

Side note: Bailey and author, N'Jhari have a unique bond. It turns out that Bailey's mom was N'Jhari's 1st grade teacher, Mrs. Beth Rhodes. Even more unique on the day N'Jhari was scheduled to have his first bone marrow biopsy, Bailey was in the next bed over getting prepped for another round of Chemo in the Tampa General Hospital, Children's Day Hospital. Although N'Jhari was plenty out-of-it from the Anesthesia, Mrs. Rhodes noticed N'Jhari and his mom (who was worried sick about unknown results) and was quickly comforting to both mom and N'Jhari… And I'd say, "we've been in friendship, family and fight ever since." Forever, One Poke, Two Pokes, Three buddies…On a mission! Bailey Rhodes is a student at her dream school, The University of Florida in Gainesville, Florida and loving college life with an infectious smile despite an occasional 'One Poke, Two Pokes, Three…'

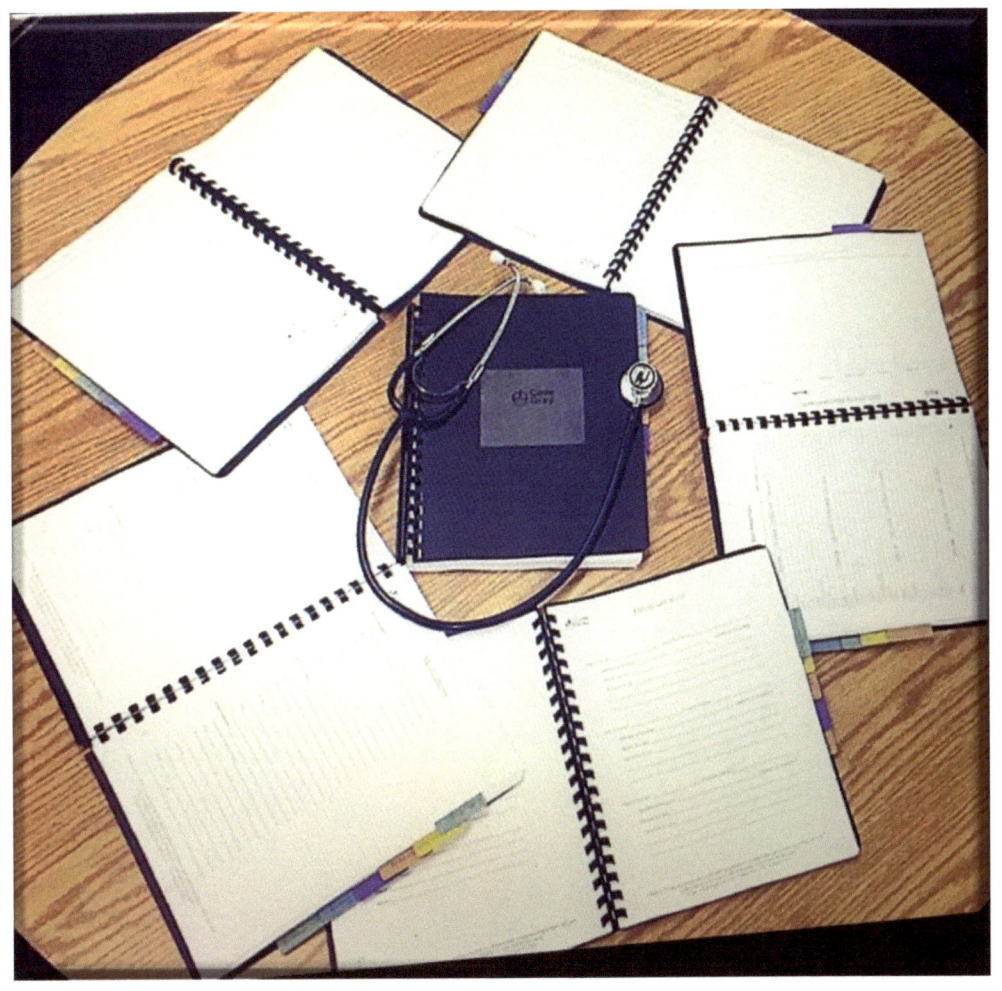

Code Blue, Code Orange… If you want to live, call Code Gray!

INTRODUCING A JUGGERNAUT…

One Poke, Two Pokes, Three

MEET THE JUGGERNAUGHT

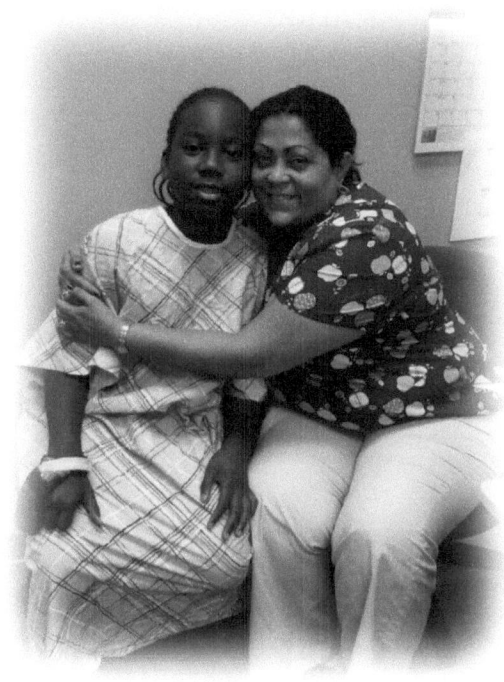

The room colorful enough for any kid, I.V. poles disguised, as giraffes while the puke canisters looked more like peppermint striped popcorn buckets. The flat screen TV's would certainly help pass time if the Benadryl didn't kick-in too soon. The "Treatment Room" is what the sign above the entry way read and despite looking like the entrance of a Chuck-E-Cheese somehow, I knew it wouldn't be fun and games. They stamp your hand; give you tickets to trade for a treat or toy without ever putting a coin in a machine. However, no treat or toy will ever make you want to comeback; certainly, I'd give back the toys and treats not to have ever taken a seat on the cozy reclining chair. A nurse says, "Here sweetie this blanket will help keep you warm," fact is I was sweating bullets out of fear. I smiled and said, "thank you." As the fear swelled inside of me, I could feel the weight of my clothes as if I had just

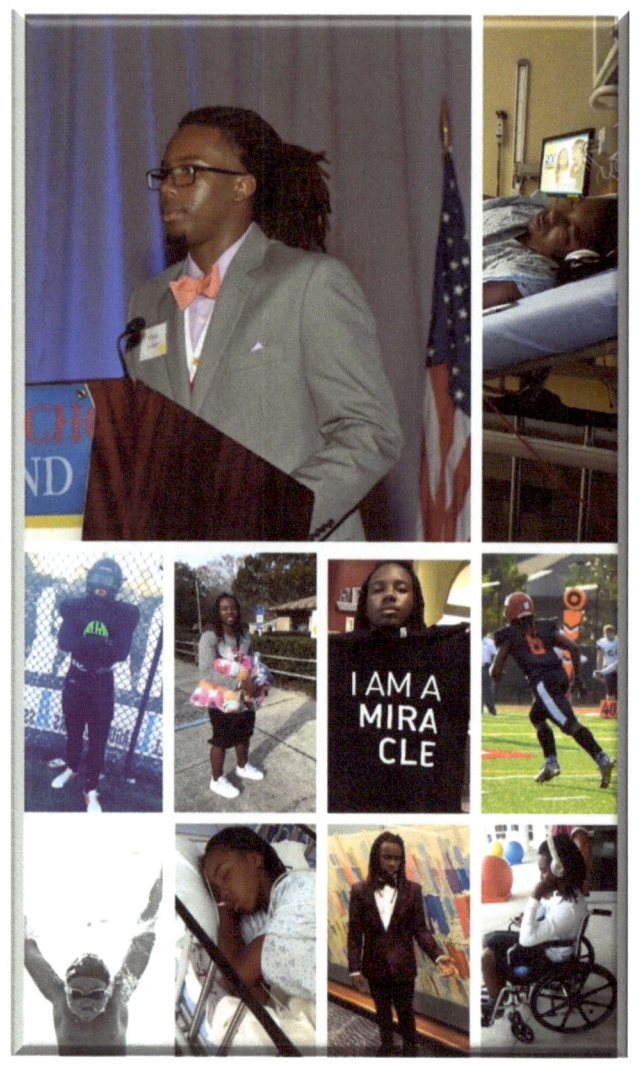

swum my best 50-Freestyle. Before agreeing to treatment for Idiopathic Autoimmune Juvenile Defects to give me a better quality of life, I watched patient videos, spoke with nurses, doctors, and scoured the Internet. I am not sure what I was hoping to find, I just searched and asked as many questions as I could think of even those that I couldn't find the words to ask somehow, I got the information I needed to help me move forward and feel better. With every trip to the operating room for joint injections, I asked more questions…I researched this thing attacking me with a name longer than most at that age could spell as if it were my dissertation. I wanted to know about the chemo-drugs, immunotherapy, fog brain, and side effects. Would the treatments be worse than the multiple autoimmune complex symptoms? Would I lose my hair with Methotrexate (chemo-drug)? Would I be dependent on crutches or a wheel chair if I chose to forgo these treatments? What would my friends say if I started to look different? Learning to research and ask questions help build confidence and help shape my character today. Instead of accepting what was told to me, I went looking for answers that I could understand. I felt in control…I felt strong. The physical strength of being a competitive swimmer started to transcend into mental strength. With a mental strengthening came calm and confidence, that this will be a temporary situation. With each trip to the "treatment room" I relaxed more, even helped to calm the fears of other kids. I laughed and kept calm so other kids would too.

When doctors told me I'd never be a competitive athlete, instantly, I felt life drain from me. After a quick blink of my eyelids, I gained composure and made a decided that report was not for me. Thus, I verbally handed it back and said, "Thanks, but no thanks doc." The juggernaut spirit in me refused to be sidelined in life. I played harder, swam faster, trained smarter… I refused to give up! I refused to let anything stand in my way. Thus, I smiled when I stepped-up on the blocks and made my Junior Olympics cuts in both Freestyle and

Breaststroke events... Not once, but twice! I smiled even wider when they said, "No contact sports, no football for you, kid!" I stepped into my bright red cleats, slid on my #40 jersey and shined as a tight-end and wide-receiver in both the Turkey Bowl and Christmas Bowl. Today, sporting different colors and a #6 jersey, I have hopes of working hard in school and on the field in college.

You see, yes, I loss some hair but it grew back. Yes, some days I looked like a zombie...I avoided mirrors. Yes, I gained weight and watched it disappear just as quickly. Yes, I wear compression socks but the "Kool" ones. Yes, I was like a kid's toy, a yo-yo. Yes, I was an immunosuppressed-juggernaut. Yes, it put a fear in me never experienced. Taking control, facing my fear with knowledge helped breakdown that fear. This is why I know my future will involve research. I know, asking questions, doing research arms you with knowledge and with knowledge the power to overcome any fear. Today, I am happy, healthy, physically, mentally strong... ready to take on any challenge.

A **juggernaut,** just not immunosuppressed!

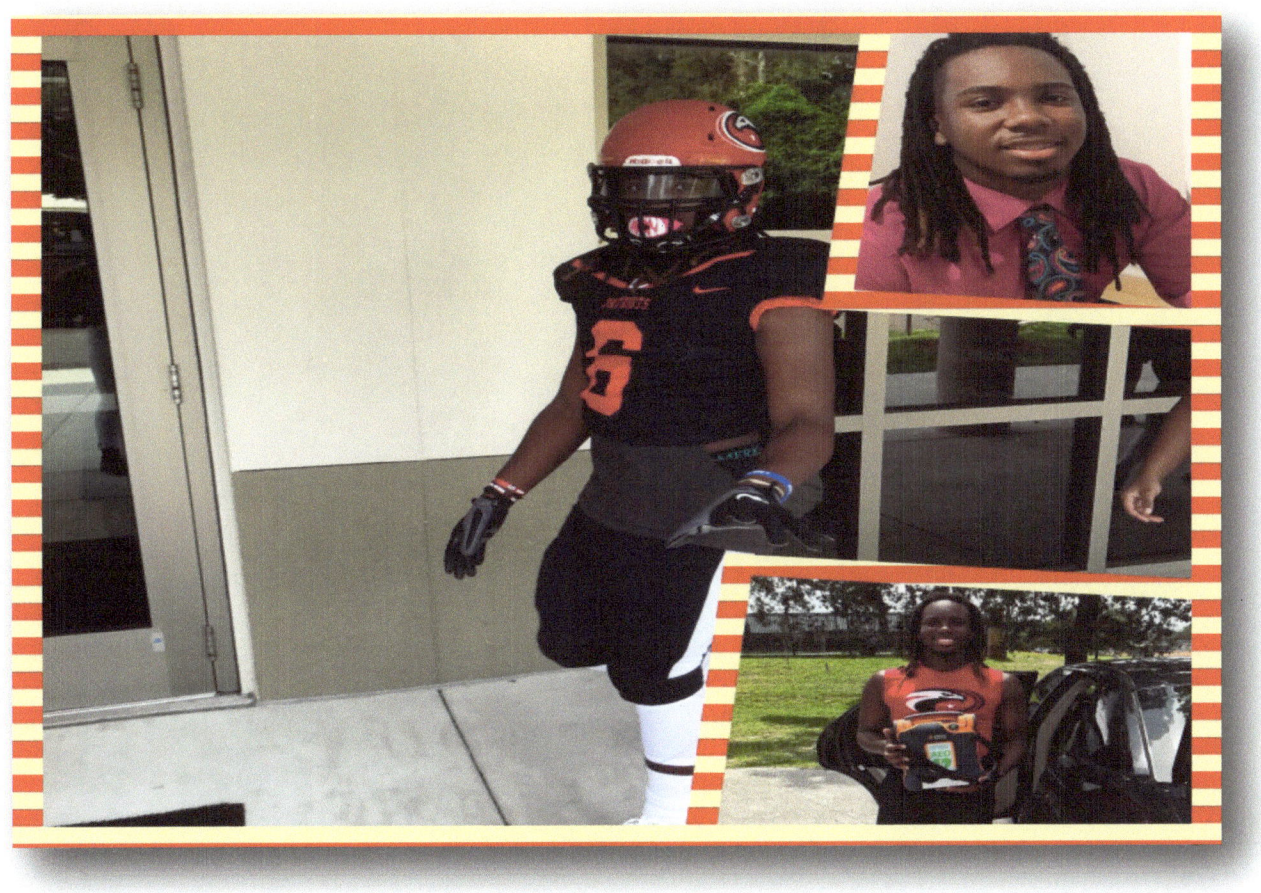

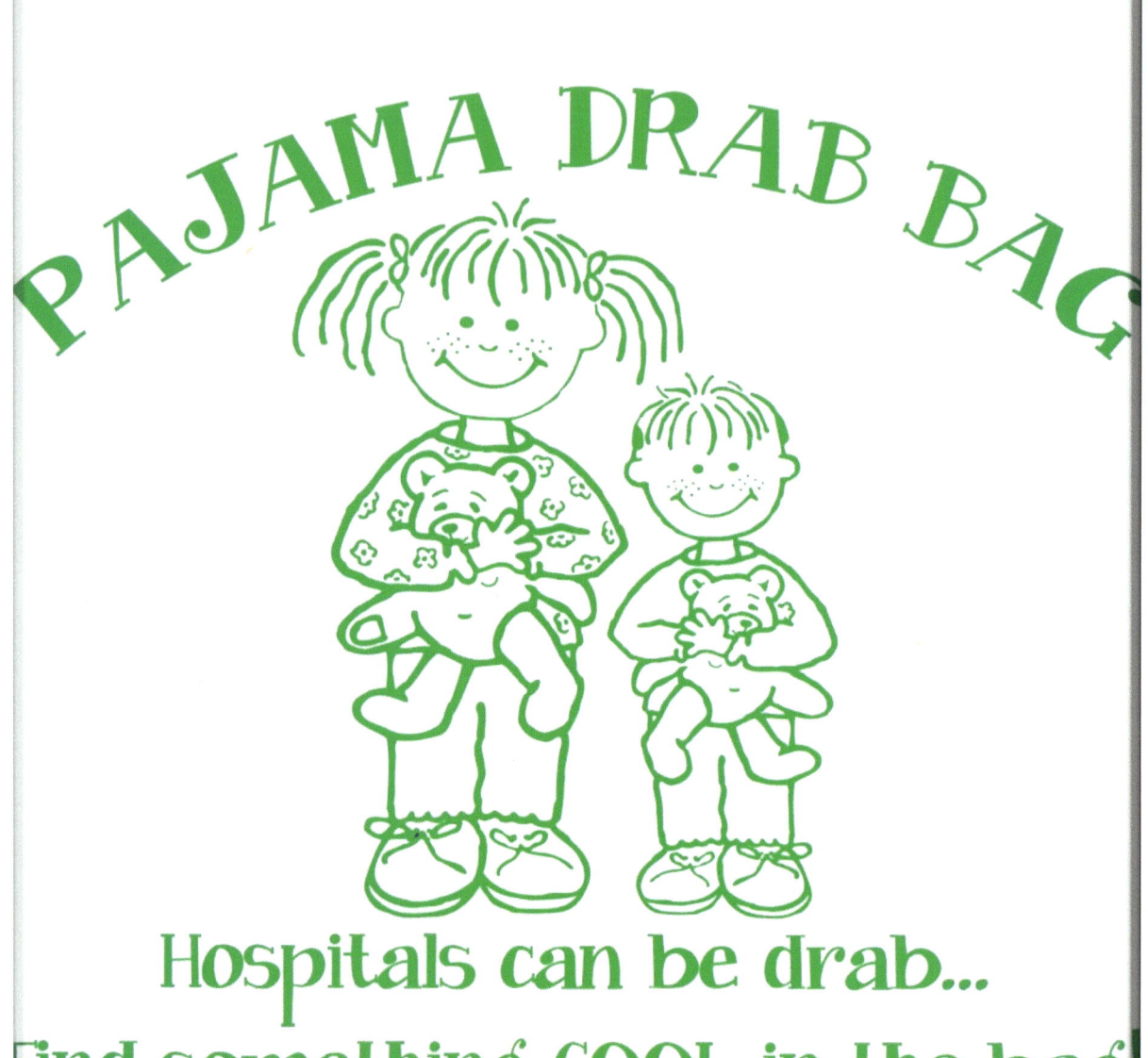

ABOUT THE AUTHOR

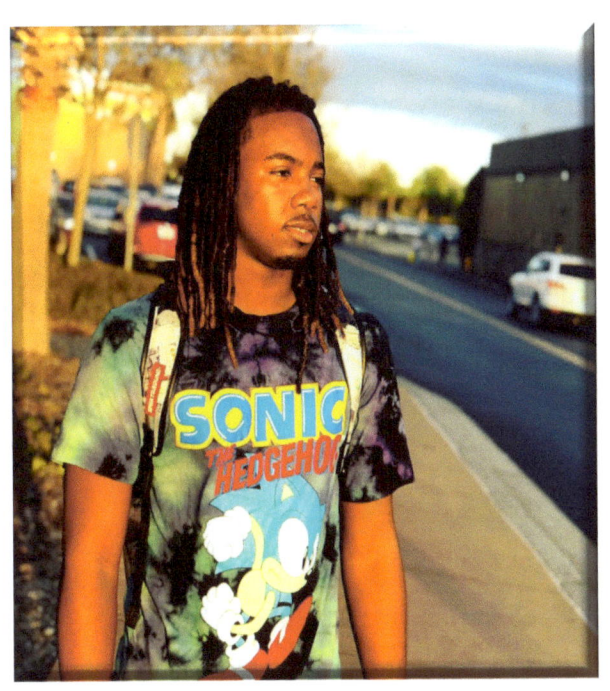

I am a 15-year-old Eagle Scout and currently a Junior at Carrollwood Day School International Baccalaureate World School. I have lived in Tampa most of my life after relocating from Chicago at 5 years old. I have a goal of earning all 138 BSA Merit Badges. I am one MB away (Bugling) from my goal… Proving to be the most difficult of all for me (this could be due to me being a lover of string instruments, bass guitar). Recently, I received the VFW Eagle Scout of the Year Award for the Florida State Department. My favorite subject at one point was math, but now I am engulfed political science, psychology, and all that peaks curiosity and debate. I also love creative writing with a flair for poetry. Last year, I had the joy of publishing my 1st book, *Revelations@13: The Compilation."* One day I'll delve into Forensic Science/ Psychology who among other things who among other things writes well. My extracurricular activities include football (Running Back and Defensive End), Swimming (Freestyle/Breaststroke),

Guitar, and Lacrosse. I enjoy the study of foreign languages and culture with special interest in Mandarin, Latin, and recently, Spanish. I have hopes of exploring China, Indonesia, and Spain. I love helping others and working in groups to solve a problem or to create something new. Having spent time in hospitals growing up, I began a project called *"Pajama Buddy Voyage & Drab Bags"* for hospitalized kids battling chronic illnesses such as pediatric cancer, autoimmune diseases, and many others, which has donated over 4,500 "goodie-filled" custom backpacks across the country in addition to, China and Germany. Being a fan of cool socks and the confidence I get from embracing my own style, I began *"KoolSox4KoolKids."* This "Kool' mission donated over 2500 pairs of "Kool Sox" to kids of Children's Home Society including The Joshua House and other group homes catering to children in situations beyond their control.

I seek out opportunities to give back to community including helping to train people in CPR/First-Aid/AED. I have donated several Automatic External Defibrillators to youth sports organizations in the Tampa Bay Area. Most recently, I donated AED's to the Carrollwood Saints Football and Cheer and Fair Oaks Rattlers Football and Cheer. I am passionate about saving young athletes from Sudden Cardiac Arrest. I advocate heart-screenings not just sports physicals for students and youth athletes. I support organizations who fight hard for young hearts including Parent Heart Watch, Saving Young Heart Foundation, Justin Carr Wants World Peace, and the Greg Moyer Foundation. I humbly accepted the 2017 Youth Advocate Champion of Heart at the 12th Annual National Parent Heart Conference. On my journey, I have been blessed to have been awarded a 4-Year Florida Prepaid College Scholarship from Gov. Rick Scott and Volunteer Florida during the 2014 Hispanic Heritage Month Essay Contest. I was selected as a participant in the 10th Class of Disney Dreamers Academy. A long sought-after goal was being a named a Carson Scholar through the Carson Scholarship Fund. I am proud to announce that I am a 3 X Carson Scholar. In 2015, I was selected as Florida's Top Youth Volunteer by the Prudential Spirit of Community Awards in which I earned a monetary award and a trip to the Nation's Capital. That same year, I had the honor of being selected as the 10th Lightning Community Hero by the Tampa Bay Lightning Foundation where I had the honor of donating $50,000 to support 5 organizations including BSA Troop 142, The Paideia School of Tampa Bay, The Joshua House for Children, Haley's House for Veterans, and Shriners Hospital for Children. As a Boy Scout, I had the honor of being selected as a Delegate to deliver the

2015 Boy Scouts of America Report to The Nation where I addressed Former President Obama in the Oval Office along with addressing members of Congress. As I am writing this closing piece, I just received a call from the U.S. Army All-Pro Football Hall of Fame in Canton, OH telling me that I have been selected as a Finalist for the 2018 U.S. Army All-Pro Football Fame Excellence Award. You can believe, I am beyond grateful and excited.

I live my life with a quote from Walt Disney at the forefront of my walk, *"Whatever you do, do it well. Do it so well that when people see you do it they will want to come back and see you do it again and they will want to bring others and show them how well you do what you do."* Whether I choose to be Forensic Scientist or Biomedical Engineer, I will be the best that I can be while being a responsible, caring, loyal contributing member of this great nation for all to see.

"May you laugh until you pee your pants and cry 'til you smile"
~N'Jhari Jackson

"When it really matters, there's a Juggernaut in all of us...
Can't stop, won't stop"
~N'Jhari Jackson

Juggernaut (n): a massive inexorable force, movement, or object that crushes whatever is in its path; extremely large and powerful force that cannot be stopped.
~Merriam-Webster Dictionary

www.ingramcontent.com/pod-product-compliance
Lightning Source LLC
Chambersburg PA
CBHW040410220526
45473CB00004B/1194